PRUNE JUICE COCKTAIL

A RECIPE FOR AGING WITH GRACE

BY

GEORGIANA K. KELLER

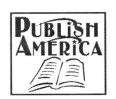

PublishAmerica

Baltimore

ISBN: 1-4241-7737-5
PUBLISHED BY PUBLISHAMERICA, LLLP
www.publishamerica.com
Baltimore

Printed in the United States of America

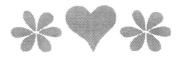

ACKNOWLEDGMENTS

How does one begin to thank so many people who gave of themselves to share a dream and make it come true? My words are inadequate, but my appreciation is sincere.

First, I will always consider the day I met Marian Frailey to be a special blessing in my life. You allowed me into your heart, Marian, to see the beautiful person you are, and to learn of the gifts of aging that you have gathered on your journey of life. You truly have been blessed to be a blessing to others.

Special thanks to Vivian Strunk, Linda Shaw, and Michelene Rich, for reading the first manuscripts when they were just an idea.

Thank you to David Zinman. Your creative writing class at Coastal Carolina gave me back my voice and allowed the dream to become a reality.

Thanks also for the patience and encouragement of the members of our writing class: Peg Slinger-Twyman, Judy Campbell, Nancy Edelman, Gloria Spivey Flecker, Gail Ritrievi, Kjersti Pratt and Sue Pearson. You helped me to believe in myself and your suggestions helped bring ideas from the heart and mind to the page.

And finally how do I thank the special person with whom I share life? You are always there, Bill, with a word of encouragement, a solution to a computer crisis, a helping hand. You truly are "the wind beneath my wings."

TABLE OF CONTENTS

PROLOGUE

From the moment we are born we begin to age. Tales of earliest times remind us that we humans have searched for the elusive fountain of youth hoping to avoid old age. Finding no eternal youthful waters, we began exploring other vistas for a magic formula, some secret ingredient that would at least make aging a more delectable dish to savor.

How does one peer into the mirror each day and conclude that aging is something beautiful? How does one accept changes and limitations and still feel life is meaningful? Is there really a secret ingredient that can be stirred into the broth of life to make it richer and more satisfying?

Several years ago, God sent a wonderful gift into my life in the form of a new friend, a truly beautiful person, Marian Frailey. Through many wonderful visits, I was blessed to learn about a rich and full life, but I learned much more. I was privileged to listen to wise insights into the aging process from one who has experienced over ninety years of journeying through life.

That is how Grace came into existence. Grace, although a fictional character, shares the wisdom of my friend Marian and others who in the winter of their lives shared with me their thoughts and feelings.

Grace is a lovely, sensitive ninety-year-old. Overcome with losses and finding her world confined to the walls of the room in an assisted living facility, she struggles to find the luster in those years some call golden. Flashbacks of life now washed down with "prune juice cocktails" give new meaning to wrinkles and gray hair. Hope replaces depression as Grace, known for her delectable culinary creations, reflects on her life and creates a new recipe—a recipe for aging.

If you are reading this book, then perhaps you too are searching for a new perspective on aging. What new flavors will be added to your life if you try Grace's recipe?

Chapter 1
CHEERS!

The soft spring breezes gently rustles the blind on the window of my room. I turn to look at the courtyard dressed in spring blossoms when a gentle knock comes to my door.

"Grace, it's time for your cocktail."

Ah, yes! Cocktails! I remember the days when my dear husband Bob and I enjoyed our cocktails. Before dinner, we would stretch our weary bodies into our recliners and talk about the day while sunlight danced off the crystal glasses.

Now my cocktail comes in a plastic cup. Its flavor is prune juice. And I do my reflecting in the bathroom!

Yes, my life has changed. Seeing my wrinkles, white hair and unsteady gait you may feel sorry for me. That's okay. I often feel sorry for myself too, but not for long. Since I've moved into this assisted living facility, I've found a new perspective on aging.

It hasn't been easy. I've struggled and clawed to get where I am today. But I have survived. I'm even starting to enjoy prunes. After all they're just plums with wrinkles!

Wrinkles! Judging from the ads shouting from my television you would think they are a curse. A "zitful" gift from years of living. I thought that too until recently.

The other day as I was doing my daily reflecting on "the throne," I had a regal thought. Maybe what I've learned about growing older could help someone else. I've always loved helping others. Just because I'm now living in an assisted living facility doesn't mean that I can't do some assisting myself! I thought about the best way to share my thoughts with others, and that's when it hit me! Why not create a recipe for aging?

Recipes have always been my special friends. While others were reading steamy romance novels, I was reading how to steam broccoli. Finding the perfect recipe was like going on a treasure hunt. I loved searching for the meatloaf that made you think of home, the classic covered dish casserole, and the dessert that would make chocoholics beg for more.

My husband said that my hobby was collecting recipes, and he was right. Cookbooks seemed to beckon to me wherever I went. Friends and strangers who collected special recipes for church and school fundraisers knew that I was a sure sale. Volumes describing the local cuisine from Alaska's streams to the cotton fields of Alabama were a prized possession. So what if I didn't live near a salmon stream or an okra field.

Each year I would add to the collection until shelves were sagging under the weight of my treasures. My cookbooks stood like a waiting army ready to be called into action. Next to them were stacks of cards filled with special instructions from friends for creating delicious dishes and lasting memories.

Armed with my recipes, I could create masterpieces with Cool Whip and Jell-O! But my favorite dessert was watching my family and friends enjoy my creations and asking for more.

As the years went by, I found that I turned more and more to my favorite recipe friends. The trusted ones who had joined me at the dining room table for years. There was a sense of warmth and happiness about creating something that my family had enjoyed. I guess that is what people mean about comfort food.

Most of my collection of cookbooks and recipe cards had to be given away when I moved here to Piney Grove. They could have filled a room by themselves, and my daughter said we were not paying room and board for them. I managed to salvage some of my favorites, and cram them into a box under my bed.

Some day I'll organize them and make a cookbook for my granddaughters. Then when I'm gone, and they make one of the dishes, they will think of me. Even though passing on my luscious pumpkin cake recipe is like passing on a part of me,

I'd rather pass on something even more satisfying—my recipe for aging.

It's taken me over ninety years to perfect it. If you would like to try it, you'll need some special ingredients from the pantry of living. But first I must tell you a little about my life and how I came to write my recipe...

Chapter 2
THE BROTH OF LIFE

Like a jet racing across the horizon, my ninety years of life have sped by, but you wouldn't find any mention of them at your local library. Most people would think my original recipe for living was pretty bland, but I know that each of the stages of my life held its own magic.

The carefree days of childhood were spent exploring a world bounded by my parent's love and concern for my safety. Lazy afternoons spent reading under the old embracing apple tree blended into evenings sparkled with the light of fireflies trapped in a glass house. I didn't have many friends, but bugs and butterflies and crickets spun webs of wonder into my days. Without television and video games, my grandchildren would probably find these days boring, but I found them to be wonderful appetizers of life.

As a teenager, I danced on the stage of life. Spending hours in my room I would pour over fashion magazines and dream of being the person I thought my girlfriends were becoming. I longed to fit in with them—to be accepted as their friend. We giggled as we shared our dreams of future dates. It didn't matter that the boys in my class only thought of slaying football demons. I knew that somewhere out there was my handsome prince and that he would appear at just the right moment to whirl me away to new adventures.

As a young woman, my prince arrived, not on a white charger, but in an old white Chevy that charged into my driveway. Rumbling through the streets of town to the movies or a dance, I not only passed new avenues in town, but in my life as well. Living took on a new zest. My senses came alive! Sunshine brightened. Moonlight softened. I ate from the buffet of life and was satisfied.

After Bob and I were married, I thought life was perfect, until the children came to show me that life could be even more beautiful. The golden curls of a darling little girl and the dark brown eyes of a strong son brought us new joy and responsibilities and we began to mix our own unique broth of life.

Thinking back to those busy days, I realize there never seemed to be enough time to savor that broth. Cleaning house, doing laundry, cooking meals, transporting kids—I was so busy doing the chores of living that I hardly had time to live.

And then, just when I thought I had finally found the perfect recipe for our life as a family, Kay and

Bobby were gone. They each found wonderful soul mates with whom to share life and they left our home to start homes of their own. I barely had time to feel sorry for myself though, for two beautiful cherubs called granddaughters invaded our lives with laughter and joy.

Bob retired and we settled into a lovely routine. We would do our daily chores, take an afternoon nap, and always stop before dinner for a cocktail and a chance to talk over the day. There were friends to meet for lunch, shopping with the girls, and evenings filled with friends and laughter. Life was good!

And then it happened! Friends who had always been here to share our life disappeared. Illness took them to hospitals, nursing homes, and finally funeral homes. Bob and I clung to each other as we entered this new phase of our lives. We searched our recipe that had served us so well over the years and wondered why the broth of life was now so thin and flavorless.

The kids thought we should move into a small cottage on the campus of a local assisted living facility where we could take it easy. After all, we were in our eighties they said. We should be able to enjoy life, not have to worry with a big old house to clean and a yard to mow that now seemed a lot larger than it used to be. So we agreed. We began to pack and I discovered the taste of moving day stew...

Chapter 3
MOVING DAY STEW

I remember packing for the move. I tried not to grieve for the loss of our house even though waves of details were crashing over me. As my salty tears splashed on the boxes and piles of newspaper, I tried to persuade myself that this move was the best choice for Bob and me. We had reached the stage in our lives where we needed help. It was time to move to a smaller place where we could be surrounded by folks who could help us with our needs. Yes, it was time to add "assisted living" to our address.

After a few lectures to myself, I was ready, or so I thought. I knew that all of our possessions from the last fifty years would never fit into our new home. Our furniture had filled and graced an eight-room house and made it a home. Overstuffed chairs hugged our tired bodies. Our beautiful cherry table and chairs were honored guests at mealtimes. Lamps of all shapes and sizes brought a warm glow to our home on cloudy days and dark evenings. Each piece of furniture was like an old friend with whom I could share stories of a life well lived within these walls for fifty years. What would happen to those ingredients of living?

It brought me joy when Kay and Bobby wanted some of the furniture and some of the decorations from our walls. The granddaughters wanted china and crystal, and the knickknacks they had treasured as children. But what about the things that no one in the family wanted? The thought of throwing them away or selling them at the auction sent a stab of pain through my heart. How could I part with the memories? What if those old framed portraits of deceased family members that no one wanted found their way to the walls of Cracker Barrel?

Memories etched in knickknacks, framed in pictures, sewn into quilts. How do you let go? It's so final. Your mind knows that it's time to move forward but your heart clings to the past and longs for the change to go away and for the happy times to be here again. You wish for the days and years to be frozen in time.

And then there was the house. I thought that I would feel no sadness about leaving the house. The old drafty place was certainly getting to be more than I could handle. Everyday tasks that used to bring pleasure now brought the reminder of arthritic hands and knees that turned the tasks into chores.

We sold the house. A family with two children became the new owners. It made me happy to know that the old house would once again hear the laughter of children echoing through her halls, and that a new pot of life's broth would be simmering in the kitchen.

And so, we moved out the furniture. We packed the boxes, and cleaned, and I walked through for one more time—unprepared for the feelings that assaulted me as I wandered from room to room.

Memories of birthday parties, and Christmases past, of friends gathered for an evening of games and dessert. Where had those moments gone? It's just a house I kept telling myself, but as I walked through naked rooms, and touched barren walls, I knew this was more than a house. It was also a friend to whom I now must say good-bye.

What would the future hold? I was soon to find out...

Chapter 4
LIFE IN A PRESSURE COOKER

In our new community, we found many friends, old and new. Some shared the same interests that we did, and others taught us new ones. My arthritic knees even learned to jitterbug, and I gave my Betty Crocker seal of approval to the meals we ate in the dining room. New friends to meet, new things to learn, fewer responsibilities. Moving had given our life a tasty new flavor.

But then came the day that is forever etched on my mind and heart. Cancer! Bob had cancer! The doctor might as well have given ME a death sentence too when he told me that Bob didn't have long to live. I couldn't believe it. This couldn't be happening. Not my Bob. Not the person that I shared sunrises and sunsets with for over fifty years. How could I survive without him?

I didn't let myself think about that possibility. Each day, I kept busy visiting him in the nursing care center and the hospital, but before I could even comprehend what was happening, Bob was gone.

It was a beautiful service. Everyone said how brave I was because I didn't cry. Little did they know that I couldn't. A wall of numbness held back the gallons of tears I wanted to shed. As I moved through each day like a shadow, my life seemed so empty, so hollow.

My friends tried to fill the void in my heart. They visited, called and wrote notes. They brought me soups of love and desserts of kindness, but I could not taste them. I could only swallow my grief. The rich, satisfying broth I planned to sip in my golden years was ruined with heaping measures of losses: my home, treasured possessions, good friends, and my soul mate. Soon another loss would be added— the loss of my independence...

Chapter 5
A NEW KITCHEN

"What to do with mother" was a tough question for the kids to answer and one with which I would also struggle. I was hundreds of miles from Kay and Bobby but I felt like we were living on different planets. In desperation, they decided to move me closer to Kay. Perhaps being near family would be the solution.

The move itself was uneventful. I arrived at Piney Grove, the assisted living facility near Kay, and found that she had already moved in my things and arranged them for me.

The room was bright and cheery. A large window looked out into an open courtyard of flowers and shrubs. My faithful recliner was waiting for me in the corner and welcomed me with a warm hug as I sank into its arms. A bright new bedspread covered my bed, and family members smiled at me from frames lined up as sentinels on the windowsill. My clothes found a place in my closet and even my denture case and toothbrush looked at home in the bathroom.

Kay brushed my cheek with a kiss, announced that she would see me tomorrow, and breezed through the door. It closed loudly behind her and ushered in a vacuum of silence and loneliness.

I felt panic begin to swell in my heart when the door opened and a friendly worker chimed, "Grace, I'm Pam. Dinner is ready."

Dinner! Nourishment!

Pam gently took my hand. With help from my walker, we started the journey to the dining room. Pam explained that it was the weekend and the administrator and activity director would not be in until Monday. "They will get you settled in then," she smiled.

Monday! Waiting for Monday seemed like an eternity, but for now I had to face dinner. As I ambled down the hall, I wondered what new recipes of life were served here...

Chapter 6
THE FIRST SUPPER

The hallway seemed to stretch forever as Pam and I pushed toward the sound of clinking dishes and scraping pots. The dining room was large and beautifully decorated, but I felt like an alien in a foreign land. Pam maneuvered my walker and me to a table in the back of the room. The ladies at the table were pleasant, but each had a hearing difficulty so the thought of a pleasant dinner conversation disappeared when the food arrived. I knew what a problem it was to not hear well. Quietly I explained to one of the ladies sharing the table with me that the lovely earrings she was complimenting were really my hearing aids.

Everyone seemed to enjoy their food and plates were quickly emptied. Everyone's plate except mine. My food seemed to catch in my throat. I couldn't eat. Panic replaced my hunger. All I wanted to do was escape back to the safety of my room.

When I reached my room, I quickly called Kay and told her I didn't think I could stay here. It seemed so frightening. I felt like a child who had been dropped off for the first day of school and was crying for her mother. This time though, I was crying for the reassurance that these strange four walls were going to someday feel like home.

I know Kay heard the panic in my voice and she tried to remind me that it would just take time to meet people and feel at home, but I was not persuaded. Five, six, seven times I reached for the phone just to hear her voice.

Finally, my first day ended with a blessing. The door opened and Pam came in with my sleeping pill. Sleeping pills—they added no flavor to my living. Instead, they let me escape from living. I gulped down my red and white friend and sank into the delicious slumber of unconsciousness...

Chapter 7
TRY THIS

Red pills, white pills, big pills, small pills! Having suffered from migraines and stomach disorders as a young person, I knew what a blessing pills could be. But pills soon became a problem for me instead of a blessing. They were toxic ingredients.

When I arrived at Piney Grove, my anxiety literally paralyzed me. As I tried to deal with the physical and mental limitations surrounding me, I felt like a net had been thrown over me. The memories of my past were trapping me and I couldn't breathe. I needed help. I felt like I couldn't do anything that made me leave my room for what was on the other side of the door.

In my room, there were family pictures and memories of the life I had known and loved— reminders of rich delicacies of living. I didn't want to leave my room. It was bright and comfortable. My music and TV were there. It was like a child's tree house. Small in size, but large in the peace and comfort that it provided from the real world. Like the view from a tree house, I could observe what was happening without really getting involved.

The pain in my heart soon led to pains in my stomach, head and back. I would press my trusty buzzer and ask for help in the form of a friend easy to swallow. The pills helped me become less conscious of the pain around me.

Soon my family and the professional staff knew that I needed help. Doctor appointments became my daily routine as we searched for the magic cure. Unfortunately, instead of finding a cure, each doctor added another pill or two until thirty pills found their way to my door each day.

Life revolved around my pills. I would swallow one and watch the clock to see when I could have another. If my medicine did not arrive on time I panicked and felt I had been forgotten. With cold, clammy hands I would press the buzzer and wait for help, and if the help did not arrive immediately, I would venture beyond my door looking for my friends in capsule form. Not only was I a walking pharmacy, I was drowning in the fog that the medication provided.

Finally, I was hospitalized, and professionals helped me to find myself again. I had been existing, not living. Clouds of doubts and fears had floated into my life and had enveloped me strangling out any rays of life's sunshine. I needed to feel quality of life again.

"Quality of life." That's a term I hear used a lot when people are talking about older people in places like this. "Assisted Living Facilities will add quality of life," the brochures announce, but I wonder what that means.

At ninety, being assisted with living, what is the quality of my life? What new ingredients for living can a place like this possibly give me? Will the broth of life served here in the normal day-to-day living bring any nourishment to body or soul?

Chapter 8
LET THE FEAST BEGIN

A friend once told me that "normal is just a setting on the dryer." That must be right, because days around here certainly don't seem "normal." Perhaps I should call them typical, and describe one for you.

First, I escape from the cozy warmth of my bed to face the day. I try to pick a cheery sweater to liven up my navy slacks and tie on my "old lady shoes" that are to protect me from falls.

Faithfully waiting for me in the corner of my room is my walker. We have become good friends since I have arrived. Silver in color, with black rubber wheels, it's my new limo. We push our way around corners and through halls.

My walker is also my purse. A smart looking cloth bag attached to the walker's bar carries all the necessary things I used to stuff into a smart looking handbag. Now I'm just glad the walker and bag are there to give me a hand.

Once I'm up, dressed, teeth and hair brushed, I'm ready to face "the other side of the door." After all, that's the only way to get to breakfast.

On my trip to the dining room, I look for smiling faces, but smiles are hard to find. The other residents seem sleepy and ready to eat and return for a nap. Even the girls in the dining room look like they would rather be back at home under their cozy covers.

But not me! I give my good morning wishes and try to brighten the room with my smiles. After all, breakfast is my favorite meal. How much damage can you do to a bowl of oatmeal?

Breakfast conversations are as bland as coffee without sugar. Brains seem to need time to warm up. After the usual morning greetings, questions about the night's sleep and the day's weather, silence is served with the oatmeal.

I take advantage of the silence to daydream about the day. What will this day bring? Will I have visitors? Will I have a letter from Bobby, and a surprise visit from Kay? Will a friend call? Will a new resident become a friend? There are so many possibilities for a great day.

Finally as the last spoonful of oatmeal slides down my throat, I'm ready to return to my room and freshen up before activities begin.

Reaching my walker that has been parked by the side of the room, I start down the hall to get ready for the rest of the day.

First I ask myself the question I ask each day, "What will I do today?" I amble down the hall and look at the white board where the day's schedule is posted. Besides the activities, I can find important information like the day of the week. Sometimes the days all seem to be faceless and one needs a reminder. There is exercise and cooking, puzzles and Bingo. Ah, Bingo. When all else fails, there is Bingo.

I never got the fever for hunting numbers under letters. Wonder who ever thought of this game? Perhaps a pirate stranded on a deserted island bored and dreaming of hidden gold hatched a plan for a secret treasure map. Yes, that's it, a secret treasure map of squares and numbers hidden under the code letters. Can't you just picture that weatherworn angel looking down from his cloud and laughing at the multitudes of people who meet daily to study his treasure map and receive treasures of their own?

Well, that theory of the origin of Bingo stretched my imagination, but I'm ready to stretch my muscles. I'm heading to the first activity of the day—exercise class.

As my walker and I push through the door, I find a deserted room. A thousand questions flood my mind. Did I misread the schedule? Am I late? Did I miss it? Where is everyone? I don't even see anyone to ask.

Finally Mary, the cook, enters the room. One look at Mary and the familiar blue and white cards in her hand, and I know what has happened.

Ginny, the activity director must be sick, and Mary will pinch hit with Bingo which will make many of my friends happy, but I still don't feel like going on a safari to find numbers under letters, so I'm out of here!

Chapter 9
INGREDIENTS OF LOVE

Back in the comfort zone of my own room, I ponder how to use this day. Should I write to friends? Should I call them? Should I take a walk or read?

What do I do? Nothing. I'm lonely, so I escape from activity and into the stillness of my room where I will sit until lunch.

My conscience chides me for wasting another day of life. I should be with the others in the activity room. But my mind screams, "There must be more to life at this stage than Bingo."

How would you fill your days if your world suddenly shrank to one room? How would you fill the minutes in the hours, and the hours in the day? I wish I had thought about this question earlier in my life.

From a four bedroom house to the four walls of one room. I guess that makes me an expert on downsizing. Downsizing—that's quite an experience. Just as I had struggled with possessions and memories when we sold the house, now I was faced with choosing only the things that would fit in my new one room home. Oh, Kay was right there to help me decide. I appreciated her ability to take charge when I just wanted to charge in the opposite direction. I listened to her suggestions, but when she wasn't looking, I gathered a few treasures of my own and put them in a locked box. And now they live here with me—my life in a locked box.

When we arrived at Piney Grove, my box survived the "let's get rid of this" hand of Kay when I told her it held family treasures. "Someday," I promised, "we will look at them and talk about them." I know Kay will never understand why I kept this box and its contents. She will probably think I spent my last days in frail mind as well as body. But something magical happens when I get out my locked box.

My ninety years of living have often closed the curtains on the stage of my mind where memories dance to entertain me. I need a little introduction before the memories can perform their magic in my life. The objects nestled in my locked box perform those introductions as they gently nudge me to remember. I need to remember now.

The rusty hinges squeak open and the sunlight reflects on some locks of golden hair. They're from my head. I found the locks when my mother died and I was going through her things. Mother was always intent on the job at hand and not very generous with her display of emotions. I always knew she loved me, even though I never heard the words. When I found my locks of hair, I knew I was right about her love for me. They were tucked in an envelope in her Bible and on the envelope she had written "From my angel Grace's first haircut." Knowing that mother, who was a no nonsense person, would keep pieces of my hair for over seventy years brought me a new joy I had never known. Those locks brought a voice to my mother's silent love.

Dried rose petals? Oh, I remember! They were from my first corsage from Bob. We went to the senior prom and danced all night. When I came home, my beautiful corsage of red roses and baby's breath looked like it had taken its last breath. I managed to cling to a few petals despite Mother's thorough spring cleanings, and now the withered petals remain as a treasure in my box. A reminder of a beautiful love that blossomed for over fifty years.

I didn't throw away this yellow, crinkled piece of paper either. It was my son Bobby's first love note. In childish scrawling it simply says, "I luv you, Mommy." Now how could I trash that? Throwing it away would be like disposing of a piece of me.

Then I notice this letter. Written on delicate pink stationery, it still holds the faint scent of perfume. The letter is from Kay sharing with me her plans for her future wedding. I cherish this line that says, "My deepest wish, Mother, is that John and I will share a love like you and Dad."

As I pick up each object, I'm transported to another place and time. Homemade Valentines from the kids, gingerbread Christmas ornaments that no longer smell of sugar and spice, lace sachets of rice from countless weddings, torn pages from coloring books that say "to Grandma with love." Junk! That's the evaluation most people would give to my objects, but for me they are as precious as gold. They hold the exquisite ingredient of unconditional love that has flavored my life for these ninety years.

"Grace, it's time for Bingo. Won't you come and join us and meet some new friends?"

"Just a minute, I need to put something away first."

Well, I'll lock this box, and slip it under the bed until the next visit. For now, I'll get up my nerve and invite my walker to join me for a stroll down to the Bingo game. Who knows? Maybe today I too will find a treasure. Perhaps a new friend will be waiting for me "under the N." And maybe when Kay unlocks this box someday and looks through its contents, she'll wonder why a Bingo card was in my locked box.

"Grace, are you coming?"

"Yes, as long as I can get to the other side of the door..."

Chapter 10
STRANGE FLAVORS

Some days it seems like I'm just not strong enough to get to the other side of the door. Oh, the door is not particularly heavy, although it is a little awkward to get both my friend the walker and me though it. Usually one of us gets hit on our backside.

No, it isn't the physical movement. It's the struggle between my heart and head—a struggle I face daily here at Piney Grove Assisted Living Facility.

Assisted living facility. The name is self-explanatory for this stage of my life. I do need assistance with living. I don't feel well enough to do my cooking, cleaning, laundry, and all those things that kept me so busy over the years. (I wonder how many dishes I have washed in my ninety years? How many shirts ironed; potatoes peeled...)

Now I am in a lovely building. People are here to care for my needs. Kay tells me that we are paying big bucks to have them take care of me. Even though it's a beautiful place, bright and warm and comfortably decorated, something is missing. It just doesn't feel like home. I miss my old friends.

New friends await me on the other side of the door. But do you remember how scary it is to make new friends?

At first, I worried that people might not like me, might not want to hear my stories about people they had never met, might not want to really spend time getting to know me. It was so hard to open that door and face what was waiting on the other side.

People were cordial, but they really didn't have time for me. The nurses and aides were polite, but too busy to really sit and talk.

The other residents were pleasant, but they were dealing with challenges too. Some could not hear well. I didn't feel like shouting my conversations. Some of the residents were confused and would often wander into the wrong room. Some would tell me the same story every day. I guess that's one advantage of getting forgetful—the same old stories seem new each day!

I longed for just a spoonful of friendship and each day I struggled to get to the other side of the door, hoping it would be waiting for me.

The days that I couldn't open the door, I retreated to my room and either to my locked box or my photo albums...

Chapter 11
DELICACIES TO SHARE

Photo albums. What treasures! As I turn the pages, I begin with pictures of my parents and me. Being an only child was a mixed bag of blessings. I certainly got my parents' full attention whether I wanted it or not. The expectation level was high for the only child in the house. After all when I got into trouble, there were no sisters or brothers to blame. I grew up tasting love, but always feeling like I didn't quite measure up to those adult expectations. Wonder if that's why there aren't many early photos.

Ah, but here are school pictures. At last I was around other kids. At first it was scary. What if they didn't like me? Why do I have to wear long stockings and boots when the other girls don't? Why are they drawing better than I am? I had a lot of questions as I struggled to find my identity in the nurturing walls of that one-room schoolhouse. Even though I questioned my gifts and abilities, I became more confident as wonderful friends encouraged my growth. These smiling faces from the pages of my memories remind me that life was changing for me.

Lucky for me that I turned both this page and the page in my life, as a wonderful new friend appeared. Yes, here's my favorite picture of Bob. I thought he was the most handsome fellow I had ever met. Just as the song says, he swept me off my feet and into a new world of love. Soon I was posing for these gown pictures. First a prom gown and then a wedding gown. And look at those babies! Stacks of pictures of the kids. Babies, toddlers, Halloween costumes, starry-eyed little ones nestled on Santa's lap, school events...

Looking through photo albums is like attending a banquet of life. Reminders of people, places and events make up the main courses. I feast on the joys of holidays, the passing years of birthday parties, the new beginnings of weddings and baptisms. I drink to each generation as they pass on the cup of life.

But like all banquets, I need to share the bounty. With excitement coursing through my veins, I extended an invitation to Myrtle my friend next door to come and feast with me. I was not prepared for what happened...

Chapter 12
A SPLASH OF VINEGAR

I was so excited. Myrtle said she would love to come to my room to see my albums. I looked forward to a wonderful afternoon. An afternoon of sharing my memories and reliving them as I explained each picture, and resurrected it from the flat page of the album to our mind's eye.

I relished the thought of sipping from the cups of memories and sweetening the day. Instead, my day turned sour as though Myrtle poured a large bottle of vinegar into my cup.

If you had been in my room, you would have heard a conversation that sounded something like this:

"Myrtle, let's start with the latest picture of my family."

"Oh what a lovely family. Who is that attractive lady?"

"That's me."

"You! That can't be YOU! Have you changed that much?"

Have I changed that much? That is a good question. Myrtle doesn't need to remind me that I am growing older. Every morning when I look into the mirror, I wonder who is looking back. It sure doesn't look like me. Where did those wrinkles and age lines come from?

Wrinkles and age lines the marks of years past. Fretful nights when the children were sick or late coming in from a date. Wrinkles of worry when Bob was so sick and the doctors couldn't guarantee his recovery.

Those wrinkles are not all from hard days. Wrinkles come from laughter too, and there were many days filled with laughter. I love a good joke and Bob would always double over when I told him one. He thought I should be on stage!

I never made it to the stage, but I did have fun staging some jokes. Getting together with my family always gave me a good opportunity especially when we played our favorite board games. A winning strategy for me was to pretend to go to the kitchen or the bathroom. Instead, I'd really go to look up the answer to the question. Pretty tricky, don't you think? It brought a laugh to all.

Laughter filled my room again this afternoon. After I got over the initial shock of discovering that I looked a lot older than the photos, Myrtle and I spent the afternoon drinking in the stories behind the photos. Laughter echoed off the walls.

Laughter! What a wonderful ingredient to add to life's broth. It felt so good to laugh and to realize that I can still make people laugh. In fact, aging has taught me to laugh at myself. That's a lot harder to do, but I seem to be getting more material lately!

The other day, my son-in-law informed me that I had my shoes on the wrong feet. I just told him that it didn't matter because I have narrow feet!

What if I joined "the wrong room club" the other day. It's not my fault that all the doors look the same.

I've read in the Bible that laughter is good medicine for the soul. Wouldn't that be a good pill? Laughter pills. I could make a fortune around here. Well, maybe I'll just dispense them without charge. After all, I have the idea that the residents are not the only ones who need to add laughter to the broth of life...

Chapter 13
SPOONFULS OF LAUGHTER

Yes, I can tell that besides the residents, the staff could use some heaping spoonfuls of laughter. For many of them, life must seem like a griddle that always has them sizzling with activity.

Leaving their homes and the needs of their families, they arrive here to the sound of the buzzers of needs. Buzzers for medicine and help with a bath. Buzzers that beg for someone to come and sit awhile and share stories.

Meeting all the needs of the buzzers usually has the staff moving through the halls as though chased by an invisible monster, but some days a soft knock grazes my door and a "Susan" will appear. She asks how I am and if I need anything, but I know that what she really wants to do is sit and talk to me. I listen in anticipation of wonderful memories from my early life recaptured through her stories. Instead, she tells me about her sick child, her cross words with her husband, her feelings of exhaustion.

It's then I realize one of life's truths. Susan and all the Susans of my world have the same needs that I do—the need for someone to listen—the need for someone to say words of encouragement and appreciation—the need to have someone lift life's burdens. These needs are not characteristics of old age but the needs of every age.

Well, I'm not too old to help. I remember reading that a frown is just a smile turned upside down, so yesterday I began turning things upside down. I found some jokes in a magazine I was reading and served them with dessert. It was like a miracle! Dull eyes were shining again and walkers seemed to glide back to their parking spots. The sound of belly laughs was louder than the rattle of dishes and the clinking of glasses being cleared from the tables. Nurses and residents paused to enjoy the fresh air of laughter shared with another.

Sometimes I still wonder why I'm occupying space on this planet. I'd much rather move on and let a younger person trade in their label of terminal for mine of terminated. I talk this over nightly with God but I haven't convinced Him yet that it's a good trade. Instead, I have the feeling that he still has some work for me to do down here. Each morning I peer in the bathroom mirror hoping I'll see an assignment posted for the day. Instead my wrinkled face stares back.

But perhaps my wrinkles are part of God's assignment—His reminder that I'm aging from

PRUNE JUICE COCKTAIL

within with a beauty that allows me the time and patience to offer love to others. Perhaps the wisdom of aging is in knowing that we should take the time to listen—to really listen. The wisdom to know that Jane is not really asking for a pill but for a friend to hold her hand. The wisdom to know that Susan is not being crabby when she listens to your heart. She is just wishing that hers did not feel so heavy with the responsibilities of her own family.

Yes, even at my age, I can still share that wonderful ingredient of laughter, but there are some other ingredients on life's shelf that my new friends here at Piney Grove have given to me. I've added them to my broth of life and it's simmering now if you'd like a taste...

Chapter 14
A DAB OF DREAMING

Joe is a permanent fixture in the living room of Piney Grove. Each morning, he and his walker amble down the carpeted hallway to his seat in the dining room. Joe eats, discusses the weather with those sitting at his table, and quickly makes his way out of the dining room and into the hallway. Patiently waiting for him is his favorite chair—an overstuffed blue chair that sits in the morning sunlight with its comfy arms ready to embrace him. Joe lowers his body into the chair's embrace and leaves the world around him to escape into the world of dreams.

One might pass by Joe feeling pity for this broken shadow of a younger, stronger man. Looking at Joe sleeping peacefully in his chair may prompt one to wonder what he was like when he was younger. Did Joe have a good job? Did he have kids to play catch with in his back yard? Were moonlight evenings spent on a back porch rocking to the sound of cicada and feeling the warmth of a special hand resting in his?

When I was a young mother, I would look at my sleeping babies and wonder what they were dreaming. Could they comprehend their future? Could they imagine what adventures and blessings life would hold? Could they begin to feel the warmth of love that people would bring to their lives?

Now as I look at Joe dreaming in the sunlight, I wonder what he is dreaming. Instead of the future is Joe dreaming of days gone by? Is he reliving charging up life's mountains and crossing the finishing lines of life's races? Does the smile on his face mirror the satisfaction of a good day's work, and the simple pleasures of coming home to family at the end of that day?

I too dream of the past. A friend once asked if that was painful. Perhaps for some it is. But not for me. You see, I allow only good memories to enter my dreams. Enough pain waits for me in the real world, so why invite it into my world of dreams.

Dreams! I seem to be reaching for this ingredient more often lately, but when the days are long and difficult, my dreams help me to find the strength to accept the changes that now I face.

Many have studied dreams trying to analyze them. Are they some special sign given to us? Do they warn of the future? Or are they a gift—a way for our minds to process the daily stresses of life and face the unknown. I'll leave the answer to those much wiser than I, but in the meantime, Joe and I will share the understanding that dreams are visitors arriving with an invitation to return to the special places and people that flavored our days with contentment and joy. Joy! That's an ingredient of living that I never quite understood until I met Jean...

Chapter 15
BLEND IN FORGIVENESS

"Mama, I love you." Aren't those beautiful words? My friend Jean began her story with these words. It was a lovely afternoon. Late autumn breezes were gently blowing the leaves to the ground like colored snow. As we glided back and forth in the white wicker rockers on the porch, life seemed good. The sunshine warmed my bones and my heart. I thought Jean felt the same, but then I noticed a cloud of sadness come over her eyes as she continued her story.

Jim, her son, is the one who uses the words, "Mama, I love you." She said that he always tells her those words as he leaves after each visit. Jim is a good man and Jean is so proud of him. Even though he is her adopted son, he is adopted only in the paperwork. In her heart, Jim is her own. Daily she thanks God for the day that she and her husband brought Jim into their lives to share the love of parent and child.

Just as joy and happiness come with Jim's weekly visits, sadness also comes in the reminder of a bitter disappointment in Jean's life. Jim is not an only child. There is a daughter. A lovely, talented daughter living a hundred miles away geographically, but living thousands of miles apart from Jean's heart.

Five years ago, there was an argument. One of those silly little things that two people argue over. Something so trivial, that now it isn't even important. What is important is the wall of bitterness and anger that has risen out of that argument and blocks any loving relationship that could exist.

Jean told me that she hasn't seen her daughter in five years. Five years! Think of that! Five Christmases, five birthdays, five Mother's Days—all without a card, or a phone call or a visit. One thousand eight hundred and twenty-five days without hearing the words, "I love you." Wasted opportunities to share love and respect.

I know Jean feels hurt. She remembers those sharp words that she and her daughter hurled at each other and the pain is still as intense as it was five years ago.

And I'm sure that Jean's daughter was hurt too. We mothers, as all humans, can also say words that cause pain. Words that stab the heart and scar one's memories.

It takes two to fight, to stay angry and hurt, to pretend that what has happened doesn't matter even though it does. It takes two to keep the dividing walls sturdy. But it only takes one to begin to tear down those walls. What if Jean made the first move? What if she called and said the magic words, "I'm sorry." What could happen then?

Maybe I'll just suggest to Jean that it would be good if she and her daughter had another chance to say, "I love you," before it is too late.

When is it too late? When one is found dead in bed? When one dies in a sudden car accident? Who knows? None of us knows what tomorrow may bring or even if there will be a tomorrow. Since we don't know, shouldn't we be willing to take the first step in rebuilding a broken relationship? I'm going to suggest to Jean that she blend in a little forgiveness to her life's broth.

She did it! Jean turned down the heat that had allowed her anger to boil, and added those three tiny words that can bring flavor back to life.

The walls that Jean and her daughter had built up between them came tumbling down. It was such a little thing that had divided them, and kept them from enjoying each other all those years.

The difference in Jean was wonderful. The pain in her dark eyes gave way to a sparkle that radiated joy. She wheeled down the halls with new vigor, and even the wheeze of her oxygen tank seemed to hum with contentment.

You've probably noticed by now that I have been saying, "was." That's because Jean died last night in her sleep. The nurse went to waken her for breakfast, and found her lying peacefully with a smile on her face.

Some would say Jean's death was a tragedy, but I think a greater tragedy would have been if Jean's life had ended with anger instead of forgiveness and love.

Thinking about Jean and her daughter makes me think about Kay and me. We don't always see eye-to-eye either. I hate the silence that envelops the room when we have an argument. Angry words that hurl through the air like daggers; feelings bruised by thoughtless comments; my self esteem stripped from my very being.

My mind rewinds our arguments and the angry words make me determined to wait for Kay to apologize. After all, I'm the mother and should be respected. Then I think of Jean and remember the look of peace and contentment I saw in her eyes. A look that resulted not from being right but from being strong enough to forgive.

Jean let me taste the ingredient of forgiveness, and now I add it to my broth. It tastes better, but it still needs something—maybe the ingredient I borrowed from Dan…

Chapter 16
A CUP OF COMPASSION

"I can't believe that is the same man." Those were Mary's words at breakfast this morning. Dan had arrived for breakfast but stood in the doorway of the dining room with a confused look on his face. It seemed like just yesterday that he had arrived at Piney Grove. A short man with silver hair and a golden smile, Dan would love to sit with us ladies serving us stories of his family and friends. We would love to see his eyes twinkle with the memories of life.

Dan also loved to sing. When we gathered on Sunday afternoons for our weekly worship services, his rich tenor voice would float through the hallway bringing others to the room to search for the source of such beauty.

I really don't know what happened. One day Dan was fine and the next day he was a shell of the man we first met. He seemed to have trouble remembering how to find his room. He lost his glasses and never could remember where his daughter was and why he was here. An expressionless face soon replaced his beautiful smile. The once sparkling eyes turned hollow as they searched for some recognition of person or place.

A visitor to Piney Grove may feel sad at seeing Dan. The hollow, staring eyes, the confused wandering may stir feelings of pity. To those of us who knew Dan when he first arrived, there is the reminder of how quickly diseases may rob one of strength and reasoning. Feelings of pity, however, do not tell the whole story of Dan.

The Dan who wanders the halls with those hollow eyes, can see something that many a person with clear vision often overlooks. If Dan hears another call for help, or sees a face with sad and lonely eyes, he stops. He may sit for hours holding the hand of a troubled person, or sitting nearby to one who looks lonely. He doesn't search for the right words or give advice. He doesn't try to correct the problem or find someone who can. Dan just sits. He sits and waits with the person and for that moment the confusion and despair of his own heart is replaced with the care for another individual who sips the broth of life.

Dan has taught me to look at people through the eyes of my heart. He has given me a cup of compassion to share with those I see in need.

Needs. I've been thinking about my needs lately...

Chapter 17
ADD THE SPICE

I know that with aging I have lost much of my independence, but I still crave that ingredient of living. And so often I search in the corner of my closet for a special pair of shoes—my red shoes.

Those red shoes have been parked in the corner of my closet since I arrived here at Piney Grove. You might look at the shoes and not see anything special about them. In fact, from the cracks in the leather, the scuffs on the toes, and the worn—down heel tips, you may think that these red shoes have seen better days. You would be right. Let me tell you what I mean.

I first bought my red shoes when I was a young wife and mother. The world was my stage, and I decided that to dance on that stage I needed red shoes! I knew that a smart pair of black pumps would have been much more practical. Black pumps could walk down the aisle of the church on

Sunday morning. They could attend PTA meetings where teachers would agree with me that my children were brilliant and well behaved. Black pumps could go out to dinner on a rare occasion when Bob and I would escape for a date like in the B. C. (Before Children) days.

Even brown loafers would have been a better choice. In brown loafers, I could glide down the aisles of the grocery stores attending to the needs of my family. Brown loafers could accompany my children to the playground for a lazy afternoon in the sun. I could slip off the loafers and chat with the other mothers while our children played in their imaginary forts and castles.

Usually I was a practical housewife who felt it was my personal challenge to make a dollar go farther than the legendary George Washington. But the day that I saw the red shoes was different.

Sitting in the window of the shoe store, they seem to beckon me. They looked like an ordinary pair of red shoes. They were plain, no shining buckles or pleated bows. No unusual toe or heel— just a plain pair of red shoes. Ah, but that was the difference, they were red!

Red—a color that meant excitement and adventure. Red—a color that meant life and dancing. When I finally entered the store and tried on the shoes, I felt like Cinderella. Bring on my Prince Charming, I was ready!

Throughout the years, those red shoes continued to make me feel like a princess. Bob and I would float across the dance floor. I would put on an ordinary outfit to go to the annual company Christmas party. Then like fairy dust, an ordinary outfit was transformed when my toes touched the red shoes. I felt beautiful. Everyone in the room could tell someone special had just entered.

I danced to the sweet music of life until I found myself here at Piney Grove. Much to my daughter's disapproval, I insisted that the red shoes accompany me to my new home.

"Mother, those old things are ready for the trash. They have seen better days."

"Yes, they have, dear." Just like magic, I can relive those better days. Days when I danced through life instead of shuffling through.

Today, as the years have robbed my body of its youthfulness, I know that my light brown, non-slip Easy Spirits are a better choice for my foot fashion. I know that as I put on my socks and shoes, and tie up the laces, that I will be safer than in my smooth-soled, high-heeled red shoes. But what about my spirit—and my world?

My world has changed. It is not easy to trade dancing on the stage of life for a rocking chair behind the stage. I want to remember the days when I liked the image looking at me from the mirror—the days my image made me stand a little taller. The days I felt the smiles of people noticing me.

Oh, people still notice me. They notice that I'm unsteady on my feet, and they reach to steady me. They notice my walker, and they hurry to open the door. I feel their smiles again, but this time the smiles are tinged with pity. That's what I don't like. I'm still me! I still feel like me inside, even though I may not look the same. My spirit is still sturdy even if the container in which it is housed needs some repairs.

So, even though Kay keeps trying to throw out my red shoes, I keep them hidden in the back of my closet. Then, when the skies are gray, and I need to dance again, I pull them out. Slipping my feet into my red shoes, I kick the reminders of my aging into the corner of my room. Just for a few minutes, I walk with my head held high, and that look on my face that says, "Look at me world. I'm going places." In fact when I do finally leave this earth, I hope that my feet will be in my red shoes.

"Grace, it's time for your whirlpool."

"Well, I guess for now I am going places, but not in my red shoes...

Chapter 18
TOSS IN CONTENTMENT

Terror—the roaring sound of water—currents thrashing my body! I'm sure the makers of whirlpools would not want to hire me to write their advertising brochures!

If you have ever relaxed in the soothing, massaging waters of a whirlpool, you are probably confused by my negative adjectives for something designed to bring contentment to tired, aching bodies. Well, let me describe my first whirlpool.

Getting there was the first challenge. Stripped down to my robe, my trusty walker and I pushed our way down the hall. Not a big deal you might say, but for me walking two miles down the LA Freeway would have been easier. I was convinced that the slumped-over, sleeping gentlemen who are permanent fixtures in our living room woke up with X-ray vision when I pushed by. Of course, that day it seemed like everyone was watching. I didn't see the President, but he was probably there too.

When my walker and I finally arrived, the tub was not as easy to dive into as I thought it would be. The sides of the tubs were like looming mountains to be scaled. Dear Susan patiently maneuvered limbs over porcelain, and plopped me into the waters of my bath. Adjusting the jets on the whirlpool, she announced that she would be "right back," but before Susan got "right back," I felt like a prune!

The gently swirling water was anything but relaxing. Since the jets were much too strong for me, I sloshed from side to side of the tub like a piece of paper in a windstorm.

When Susan finally reappeared, she apologized for being so long. Of course other residents needed her too. And since my body had not turned completely black and blue, she found it hard to believe that I had been whipped around in the RELAXING warm water.

I guess that is just another example of perspective. Susan would have loved to slip off her uniform, get in that tub, turn on the jets, and soak for the rest of the evening. She would have enjoyed the peace and quiet of being in that room alone with only the sound of the whirling water. That sound could block out the other sound—the sound of beepers. Beepers calling for her attention. Beepers splitting her in a dozen ways. That sound could have drowned out the thought of her children at home with a babysitter while she worked as a single mom to provide for their needs.

Susan could not relax because of her responsibilities, and I could not relax because of my fears. Contentment was sloshing in front of our eyes, but we were blinded to its image.

"Let's get you ready for dinner," Susan's words echoed above the hum of the whirlpool.

Gladly I allowed Susan to rescue me from my troubled waters and dressed for dinner.

Dinner! Maybe my need for contentment will be satisfied there...

Chapter 19
DINNERTIME

Dinnertime at home was always a hustle and bustle time, but one I loved. Since I was a "stay at home mom," I had all day to plan my meal, and sometimes it took me that long. I wanted the meal to be perfect! I wanted to please Bob and the children. It made me feel good to cook a delicious meal and watch the smiles on their faces as they enjoyed each bite.

A characteristic of looking back must be to only remember the good. I know there were times when my meals were not perfect. Burnt offerings on a plate and the new recipes rejected even by the dog should also be in my memory bank.

Nevertheless, it was nice to have everyone around the table and to hear Bob and the children talk about their day. It really didn't seem like work to cook and clean the dishes. I loved doing it and I loved feeling needed. Memories of dinners in the past now make the present ones even less flavorful.

Now my walker and I push our way into the dining room. Thirty pairs of eyes greet me. Some of them smile at me and others watch to see if I remember where my seat is. If I don't, they will be sure to tell me.

But I know. I sit at the only seat that was available when I came. It's the seat that faces a blank wall. Oh, there are people on the other side of the table, but they are too sick to eat, or too deaf to hear me, so I just look at the wall.

Even if the food was good, I think the wall makes it bland. If only an exciting painting graced the wall—a sunny beach under the palms of Hawaii; a snow capped mountain in the wilderness of the Alaskan frontier; a serene garden filled with colorful blossoms and fluttering butterflies. Then my mind could wander into the scene and have dinner with the residents of the imaginary homes in the painting. But instead, the wall is blank, and so is my mind.

Reaching for the salt shaker, I wish I could have a magic salt shaker. I'd sprinkle our conversations with the spice of lives well lived and stories remembered. Unfortunately, only salt comes out of the shaker and a look around the table reminds me that most of the folks have been sleeping in the living room or in front of their TV's. When I comment on the weather or the news, they just stare or get confused.

I end up just looking at my food and the more I look, the less I like what I see. What is this meat anyway? I've come to call it mystery meat because it is a mystery to me to know what it is and how I am going to eat it. When I try to cut it, my knife bounces back.

In despair I ask, "Susan, may I have a peanut butter sandwich?"

"No, dear, you have eaten that for three nights, and now we are out of peanut butter."

"What about cottage cheese and applesauce?"

"No, we are out of that too. Are you sure you don't want to eat this Mexicali chopped steak?"

"Yes, I'm sure. In fact, I don't think, I'm hungry. I'll just go back to my room. Could you bring me toast and tea with butter and jelly for the toast?"

"Of course, darling. I'll bring it right away."

"Right away?" Ah, those are two words that now have new meaning for me...

Chapter 20
SIMMER SLOWLY

The words "right away" must be an example of different things to different people. To me, "right away" means by the time my walker and I push our way back down the hall, and I settle into my recliner, turn on the nightly news, and get comfortable, there will be a knock on the door. Smiling Susan will arrive with a steaming cup of freshly brewed tea, and two warm pieces of toast. The toast dripping with melted butter will be served on a pretty blue plate. Beside the plate will be spoonfuls of jelly to sweeten both the toast and my bland thoughts of dinner.

But in reality, I sit through the nightly news and two of the evening game shows only to remain "tealess" and "toastless." In frustration, I press my buzzer and ask for help. And again I hear the words, "We'll be right there."

Another half-hour goes by and finally the door opens with Susan's cheery voice saying, "Oh, I'm sorry, I got delayed by some of the other residents needing help getting to their rooms. Here is your tea and toast."

I look at the tray and notice a cup that is not steaming sitting next to two naked pieces of bread.

When I ask Susan about it, she says, "Oh, I'm so sorry. The tea must have gotten cold and I forgot the butter and jelly. I'll get it "right away."

"Right away." What do those words mean? Do they mean as fast as humanly possible or do they mean when I get around to it?

One lesson that aging has taught me is that when you depend on others for help, then you must know that not everyone will calculate time as you do. Years of living have taught me that time is not always measured by the seconds and minutes and hours of the clock.

That was a hard lesson for me to learn. I used to sit and stare at the clock. I would count the seconds slipping by and feel my blood pressure rise. As much as I would like "right away" to be right away, I have learned that jellied toast and steaming tea may not be the most pressing needs of the moment.

The Susans who are hired to help me often report for their shift only to learn that they are the only available person on duty that night. Beepers for tea, beepers for medicine, beepers for help getting into bed. If I were them, I'd wish for a beeper malfunction so I could have a minute of silence!

No, I no longer get angry with them. Instead, I say a prayer that God will give them strength to do their job and to see that job as an opportunity to share love and care with others.

Yes, aging has taught me more about time and patience. I'm trying to add patience to the circumstances of living in which I find myself.

But just in case you think that I have mellowed to the point of accepting less than I deserve, let me tell you that tomorrow is another day, and when it dawns, I'm visiting the head chef...

Chapter 21
THE HEAD CHEF

You may think that the head chef here at Piney Grove works in the kitchen but she doesn't. Instead she's in the director's office, for after all, she hires all the other cooks who stir the pot. She has told me to come to her anytime there is a problem, so today I decided to tell her about cold tea and naked toast.

My body may be creaking a little more and I'm not as strong as I once was. My hearing and eyesight may be poorer, but my mind is sharp and I'm here to speak for myself, and for those who can't speak for themselves.

You may be admiring my fortitude, but this hasn't always been me. At first, I was too timid to go to Julie. What if she got angry and was nasty with me? What if she told the staff to ignore me, and "take it out on me?" When you are depending on other hands to help you, you do not want to slap those hands.

I tried to convince Kay to do my battles, and she fought many of them for me. At first she was in Julie's office everyday. I know that was hard on Kay because she felt like she was always complaining. Complaining! I hate it when I complain. I feel like a teakettle steaming out negative things that are happening to me.

For awhile I decided to choose a different approach. When I couldn't eat the unappetizing food on my plate, I convinced myself that it was a good time to lose some weight and have my clothes fit a little better. Maybe I could even get a new wardrobe to match my red shoes! So what if they brought me a blue pill when I was supposed to have a yellow one? I like all colors and anyone can make a mistake. What if my buzzer was not answered for an hour? I could just watch another TV show.

Then I realized that this was not complaining. It was just helping the staff know that some things on the back burner needed attention. If I were having trouble eating the food because it was either raw, hard, or beyond words of description, then others might have the same problem. If mistakes were made in my medications, maybe they were made in others, and maybe those folks could not speak for themselves. If a buzzer was not answered immediately, it might be a matter of life and death to someone who had fallen and was lying on the floor needing immediate attention.

That is when I decided that I would not be complaining to discuss concerns with the director. I swallowed hard and marched into Julie's office.

With a firm voice, I listed my concerns adding, "I'm not paying for cold tea and naked toast!"

I was especially descriptive about the problem of unanswered buzzers. My word pictures projected bodies lying on the floor, blood oozing from six-inch gashes on foreheads, staining the light tan carpet and opening up a myriad of lawsuits. Julie's face paled, and she promised to take care of the problems "right away."

I'm sure she will. After all, if she doesn't, I too can come back "right away." And when I do, I may just tell her how I feel about the cooks...

Chapter 22
TOO MANY COOKS

Have you heard the expression, "Too many cooks spoil the broth?" Well, that could describe what's been happening in our kitchen here at Piney Grove. No, I don't mean that our kitchen is staffed with numerous cooks creating delicious dishes for each resident's individual needs. "Too many cooks" refers to the constant change in the kitchen staff here.

I always know when it happens. Just when I think the food is improving, strange things begin to happen. The oatmeal becomes so runny that you don't need to add milk. The vegetables taste bland and mushy, and mystery meat finds its way back on our plates. Another clue is that each meal features sauerkraut! "When in doubt throw in the kraut" only means one thing—another new cook!

"Who's in the kitchen?" is asked as frequently as "What's for dinner?" The kitchen door seems to be a revolving one!

Oh, I know it must be a thankless job to cook for folks who live here. Some of us have dentures that don't fit or no teeth at all—we need soft things. Some of us have irritable bowel syndrome. Give us spicy foods, and we will let you know about it for days. Some of us can't see very well, and so beautiful presentations go unnoticed and unappreciated. Because many of our taste buds are not what they used to be, foods taste as uninteresting as the eighth grade novel we were forced to read. Some have diabetes, some need low fat, and some need extra protein. Besides, no matter what you try to do to make the food more appealing, you will never be able to make the dish the way our mothers did.

If I had to cook for the folks who live here, I would leave too -especially when better conditions exist somewhere else. Oh, I hear them talking:

"I can make more money at Pleasant Grove."

"I'll have better hours at Sunny Spot."

"Brighter Days is closer to my home and the kids' school."

I understand. The folks who work here have families. They have bills and responsibilities to meet. Things are expensive now and many families feel both parents must work to make ends meet. I listen with sadness to the conversations of single parents who try to juggle families and bills with basic needs like sleep.

I know I have to be realistic, but just once it would be good to know "who's in the kitchen" since Laura is now at Pleasant Grove, Chris is checking out Sunny Spot and Jack has left for Brighter Days.

Mealtimes are so important in places like this. For some of us, it's the highlight of the day. When one meal is over, we wait in the hall anticipating the next one.

Have we come full circle again? Seems like when we were first born mealtime was also the highlight of our days. Food was needed then to help us grow. Of course, babies can't tell you if mealtime means more to them than just food. I wonder. If babies could describe mealtime, would it sound like this?

"Hey, mom. Are you still there? Just checking. I need a little reassurance that you haven't deserted me. I'm not here in this strange place alone, am I? Could you just tell me it's okay? You usually tell me it's okay when I get that warm white stuff. It's nice, but what I really like is the touch of you holding me close. I like looking up at your face, and smelling your perfume. I like the feel of your pat on my back. It really does make me feel that I am important to you, and you really like having me around."

Full circle. Isn't that what we "older kids" are also saying? "I just need to know that I'm important; that you're glad I'm still here. I need to know that I'm more than a body taking up space. I need to know that it's okay, because sometimes it gets scary. Just like when I was first born, this seems like a strange place, and I'm not sure where I fit."

Knowing our special dietary needs, knowing how to make dishes taste good and look appealing is more than a job, it's an art—an art of love. I know that seeing the look of contentment in hollow eyes, or seeing a smile of pleasure on a wrinkled face does not pay the rent, but how can the value of some things be measured?

Maybe I should volunteer to help the director interview the next cook. I know what my qualifications would be: applicant must know how to cook delicious meals to satisfy varied dietary needs and be able to season each dish with love, patience, understanding, and compassion.

I'd remind the applicant that even though the wages will be minimal, the rewards of contented smiles will bring nourishment to his or her body and soul. I'd even offer an added bonus if the applicant could remain in the position until the next century!

But until I see Julie in the morning, I guess I'll just have some sauerkraut...

Chapter 23
LIFE'S INDIGESTION

I knew I shouldn't have eaten that sauerkraut! Just as soon as I closed the door to my room, I knew my old companion was waiting for me. Lately it seems as though pain is my constant companion. I've heard many jokes about old age, stiff joints, creaking bones, and aching backs. But I can tell you that these body pains are no joking matter. Neither is the constant pain in my stomach.

Pain usually visits me in the wee hours of the morning, barely allowing the clock's hand to strike midnight and usher in a new day. A sharp stabbing pain cuts through my system to let me know of his presence. It starts in my stomach but soon consumes me like a wildfire in a dry forest.

Forced to leave my bed, I find that my knees are stiff and unbending in the darkness of my room. My shoulder creaks as I reach an unsteady arm toward the lamp on the bedside table. Sitting up in my chair, I wait for the pain to move to another room down the hall, but tonight he has decided to stay with me. Throughout the hours till dawn, he reminds me of my body's deterioration. How much longer before I can't get out of that bed at all?

I ring my bell for the nurse to come and bring me a pill, any pill. Just some pills that will make this unwanted guest leave. It seems like an eternity before the door opens and Sarah comes in. Hearing my needs, she senses that my pain is more than physical. She puts her arm around me, and reassures me just like I used to reassure my children after a bad dream.

But mine is not a bad dream. It's reality. I am getting older. Knees, shoulders, and backs are etched in aches. Eyes and ears no longer bring in a clear picture of my world. The pain that used to go away with a pill now refuses to leave.

Sarah stays until a beeper sounds and another resident needs her. She too has company of the uninvited guest called pain.

When I was young, my pain was mainly headaches. I guess now in looking back on life, those headaches were often from stress.

Stress! That seems to be the buzzword today for all kinds of ailments. Magazine and newspaper articles tell about what stress can do to the body and what you should do to lessen stress in your life. If you read between the lines, the best way to avoid stress in your life is not to live. Just living is bound to cause stress.

I feel sorry for young people who are working and balancing raising a family. I know what a full time job raising a family and caring for Bob was. I can't imagine doing all that and working an eight to ten hour responsible job as well. No wonder, my granddaughters, and the girls working here talk about stress and feeling exhausted. I'm sure they are getting headaches.

But back to my pain. I'm not really having headaches anymore. Now my pain seems to be in my stomach. That sharp pain that wakens me in the middle of the night robs me of activities during the day, and makes me wonder how much more of it I can tolerate.

What's worse than the pain is that there seems to be nothing to lessen it. The many doctors that Kay has taken me to see seem puzzled about what can help, or at least what can help "at my age." Ah, the famous words, "at my age."

What does that mean? Am I at the age when nothing works anymore, or am I at the age when people feel the pain is all in my head (and I don't mean a headache.)

It's even difficult to explain my pain or to find a pattern for it. Some days a certain food may agree with me, but the next time I eat it, I spend the night in the bathroom. I am happy to be invited to go to Kay's or to my granddaughter's house, but then suddenly, I have an attack, and the only trip I take is from the bed to the bathroom.

Why can't I get this pain under control? Is it mental? Am I anxious, and causing the pain? Is it physical? Is there really something wrong with me that causes the pain?

At times it seems like my pain is not about what I eat, but what eats me. Perhaps the pain I feel now is somehow related to fear. Fear that I'll be alone. Fear that no one really cares anymore. Fear that my days will be hollow and empty.

And that means that I'm making fritters again...

Chapter 24
FRITTERS

It seems as though I've been making fritters all my life. A spoon of fear, a dash of doubt. Rolled together to form a ball of emotional knots that I allowed to sizzle on the skillet of life.

When I was a child, I ate them in the dark. Cowering in my bed, they tormented me with "what if questions." "What if there's something under your bed that is going to get you?" "What if your mother and father leave you alone?" "What if Santa doesn't bring that doll?"

I didn't know they would be served at school but there they were on my lunch tray. "What if you fail the test?" "What if the girls don't like you?" "What if no one invites you to the dance?"

After I survived school and met Bob, I was sure that I had finally thrown out the recipe. But a large box of fritters were already waiting on the doorstep of my new home and life. "What if you are not a good wife?" "What if you are not a good mother?" "What if your family is killed in an auto accident and you are the only one left behind?"

Those fritters gave me terrible headaches that sent me to bed. They squashed my dreams and caused the cream of life to curdle. I would hide under the covers and pray that both the headaches and the "what ifs" would go away.

Some days they did! Some days I marched out at dawn to seize the day—just that day—and not worry about what was behind or what would lie ahead. On those days not a crumb of the fritters could be found.

I wish that I could tell you that I eventually outgrew my need for them. I wish that I could tell you that with the wisdom of aging, I quit drizzling my dishes with doubt. Instead, as I moved into Piney Grove, fritters became my steady diet especially on dark, cloudy, empty days.

"What if Kay doesn't come back from her trip?" "What if no one talks to you at dinner?" "What if you run out of money and they make you leave here?" "What if your family doesn't want you around because you're too much of a bother?"

Do you make fritters, too? Do they give you the indigestion of scary questions in the dark? Do they rob your days of sunshine and fill them with dark clouds of doubts?

I've searched for many years for the perfect ingredient that would replace the bitter taste of doubt with the rich flavor of peace and contentment. I've never really found that magic ingredient, but I have discovered something. If I spend the day caring for another, I seem to lose my appetite for fritters.

Slipping a get well card under the door of a sick resident, sharing a smile or chatting with someone whose lonely eyes meet mine seems to help me to forget my own fears. I can't do many of the things that used to fill my days, but I can do those little things of life that mean so much to another.

And since I'm no longer craving fritters, I can try and satisfy another craving—a craving for respect...

Chapter 25
A CRAVING FOR RESPECT

What are your cravings? Chocolate, ice cream, pizza? I crave respect and one place it seems to be lacking is in my doctor's office. Let me tell you what happened today.

Have you heard of the invisible man? Well, today I was the invisible woman. It started out like any other trip to the doctor. Knots in my stomach and a dull thumping in my head accompanied me down the hallway as I gritted my teeth and prepared to wait.

Loading me into the front seat of the car and my walker into the trunk, Kay reminded me not to fret about waiting. I listened patiently but in my mind I pictured the perfect trip to the doctor's office. A smiling face waiting for ME at the door with wonderful words like, "Grace, we've been waiting for you, come on in."

My daydream ended abruptly as I stepped into the office and found myself in a straight cold leather seat—cold and unfriendly as I felt. Magazines did little to help. They reminded me of delicious food my digestive system no longer tolerated and beautiful places I could no longer visit. Kay didn't want to talk since she had found an article that she wanted to read. I counted the flowers in the pattern of the carpet, and was about to begin on the blocks in the ceiling, when I heard my name. "Grace." If only I could find grace!

Much to my surprise, we entered the examining room and the doctor appeared. He smiled warmly and shook hands with Kay and me. He even noticed my red outfit and told me how nice I looked in it. I was about to tell him how much nicer it would look if Kay would let me wear my red shoes, but he had turned and I had become invisible.

He and Kay became engaged in a lengthy discussion about me. He asked all the right questions pertaining to my health. Their words batted back and forth like a ball in a tennis match:

Kay: Do you think Mother really needs that vitamin?

Doctor: No, she doesn't need that "at her age."

Kay: Does she need more tests?

Doctor: No, "at her age," why put her through that?

I wanted to scream, "Does anyone know I'm still here? Why don't you ask me what I'd like to do? My mind is still clear. I can still answer questions. Why aren't you asking me the questions?"

But before I could get the words out of my mouth, the doctor told Kay to continue the medications I was on, and bring me back in three months. Kay guided the walker and me to the door. I left the office feeling like a car that has just passed inspection. I had been looked at and evaluated, and I felt like a sticker had been stuck to my forehead that said I should last awhile longer.

I wonder how I get a new sticker—one that says "Still able to communicate." Just because I need a walker to help me go through the door, does not mean that the door to my mind is closed. I can answer questions about my own health. After all who knows better how I feel than me? I've lived with this body for over 90 years.

Well, today I kept my feelings to myself. I was a good invisible patient barely seen and definitely not heard. I watched from the outside of the conversation circle like a newly departed looking down from the ceiling. But even though I was good and did not scream or throw things, I was not good at accepting what had just happened. I had blended into the wall and out of the vision of caring because "at my age" it was easier to talk *about* me than *with* me.

Today I listened. Today I was invisible. But next time I'm wearing my red shoes with my outfit so that at least my feet will be visible as my invisible body walks out. After all, I don't like leftovers...

Chapter 26
LEFTOVERS

Mother was a good cook. Our table was always laden with delicious foods but I hated leftovers. Some people tell me that leftovers taste just as good as the first time they are served, but not to my taste buds! That's why I don't like being treated like a leftover either. I may look like I'm left over from life, but I'm not! I still want to be noticed. I still want to know I'm special to my family and friends. I want to know that I'm not a leftover of their lives pushed to the back of the refrigerator of living.

Needing to be noticed. Ah, that's a staple ingredient isn't it? As infants we cry for the milk of reassurance. As children we sob at the bruises of life yearning for loving lips to kiss away our pain. In our independent days of youth, we turn to our peers for acceptance, and we often hide our true identity in order to be identified with the crowd. Years of adulthood find us striving for those trophies of life that tell us others notice when we do a good job—that we are valuable to someone along life's way.

Yes, the need for acceptance is an ingredient that flavors the broth of life for both young and old. Now as the years have passed and I have more time to reflect on life, I realize that depending on others for acceptance is now not as important as learning to accept myself. This lesson has not been easy. Especially since my primary textbook is the mirror. Looking into the mirror reminds me of what I notice every day. The world is a lot fuzzier now than it used to be. Chairs appear in the middle of my path. Corners of doors seem to stick out farther than they used to, and definitely the newspaper and phone books are printed in much smaller print.

Oh, the joys of being young in an old body! Some days I wonder whose body this is. Who moved into my body when I wasn't looking? I feel like I've been robbed. My twenty-twenty eyesight glowing like a hundred-watt bulb has been replaced with a dim twenty-five watt substitute. My hearing always keen enough to hear the quiet whimper of my babies now has been replaced with the garbled noise of sounds I cannot distinguish. The knees that once could climb mountains of stairs each day, now have trouble bending to help me out of my recliner.

Then there's my internal plumbing. Sometimes it works, and sometimes it doesn't. Sometimes things flow through nicely and at other times there is a massive tie up! The other day the pain was really intense. I called for a pain pill to get things moving again. Imagine my surprise when I was told that I couldn't have one because taking so many pain pills was bad for my liver. My ninety-year-old answer was one that I'm sure many of my friends here would echo: "Give me the pain pill, and when I die, tell them I had a bad liver!"

Maybe leftovers would taste better if they had a new name, and maybe I could accept this stage of life in which I am now living, if I stopped to think of the new things my old eyes and ears have heard...

Chapter 27
SWEETENED WITH CHILDREN

"How are you feeling today?" That's a question that gets dispensed with my daily medications. You should have seen the look on Amy's face this morning when I told her I thought I was pregnant. Well, Sarah of the Bible was ninety when she got pregnant! Of course, now that I think about it, if I *were* pregnant again, I think I'd like to have grandchildren first.

Those of you who are parents know what I mean. With parenthood comes responsibility. There are no instruction guides attached to the bootie of that adorable little bundle you bring home from the hospital. He or she is all yours. Oh, you can read all the guides, all the books of "how to," but you will soon discover that your little one is unique, and not acting like the child described in those pages of suggestions.

Days and nights are filled with meeting the needs of your child. In the beginning you have to be a mind reader and try to interpret what the need is through the pitch and sound waves emitted from those little lungs. Soon those little lungs develop and are housed in a growing teen who makes quite clear what his or her needs are.

As a parent I asked countless questions about the decisions I was making in raising my children. Just when I thought I knew the answers the children were gone—off to make their own decisions.

Then came my first grandchild. If you are like me, it finally hits you. The awesome, raw beauty of life housed in that little pink body. Ten perfect toes and fingers—a miniature adult with countless possibilities all wrapped up in a soft cuddly blanket stenciled with lambs and violets. Why didn't I notice this in my own children?

When Kay and Bobby were small, I was so concerned that I do everything right. I read the best manuals of the day, and was worried when the children were not doing what the page for their stage of development said they should be doing. I was so busy keeping the perfect house, cooking the most nutritional meals, giving them the best educational opportunities, and entertaining their friends, that often my tired, droopy eyes at the end of the day failed to see the world through their eyes.

My eyesight improved, however, when I became a grandmother. Finally my eyes could see the world through the eyes of a child. Clouds were no longer watched for signs of rain that might spoil laundry day. Clouds were watched for dragons, and pirate ships, and all those other imaginary shapes that fluffy white clouds hold for the eye of one filled with wonder.

The wonder of life! Yes, there were butterflies and kittens, rain puddles, and dandelions. We went to the ocean in the summer and there were waves beckoning us to new adventures, diamonds sparkling in the surf, and treasures lying on the shore for us to discover.

We went to the mountains in the fall and there were gentle breezes rustling through colored leaves that fell softly into a multicolored carpet at our feet. We went outside in the winter, and in the glistening snow transformed the yard into forts guarded by powdery snowmen with carrot noses. When spring came, we watched in wonder as flowers painted the fields with color and baby robins chirped their hello to a world filled with beauty.

How blessed I am that my eyesight, now dim, was still keen enough to look at the world through the eyes of my grandchildren and great grandchildren. Their eyes have become my eyes. Now if I could only borrow their ears...

Chapter 28
MINCED WORDS

"What did you say?" seems to be a question I am asking frequently. That is, if I'm honest. Sometimes I just smile and pretend to have heard what was said. That usually gets me in trouble and I have to admit that I didn't hear what the person really said.

It's not that I'm vain about wearing my hearing aids. It's just that I wish I could hear like I used to hear without having to look for my ears in a box.

But then an incident happened yesterday that reminded me that sometimes I'd rather *not* hear what was said. Yesterday, Florence, one of the girls helping on the morning shift, used words that hurt both my ears and my heart.

I was having one of my bad mornings when my breakfast just wouldn't go down. I needed a spoonful of patience and hoped that Florence would dispense one with my morning medication. Instead she barked unkind words at me that certainly did nothing for my already troubled digestive system.

Words! They can glaze our days with compliments or blacken them with despair. I listen to the television experts telling parents how important a positive self-image is for children, and how they need to fill their children's lives with compliments and encouraging words.

Are we "older children" any different? Living with us can be frustrating too as we try to live with our limitations. Just like the little ones, we sometimes make messes for others to clean, or we cause problems without much effort. We also can find our self-images burned by words spoken without thought.

What do our words really say? Do they tell of a hurt that has lived in our hearts for years and crashes out when a word spoken in anger, frustration, or exhaustion opens the door?

Perhaps like packages our lips should carry labels: "fragile; handle with care;" and "do not open." Once our words have spewed out like an angry volcano venting the feelings hidden deep within the craters of our hearts, we cannot take them back. Like hot lava, they spread out over our days and harden the relationships of our lives.

If only we would take the time to listen more with our hearts than our ears. If only we could say those magic words, "I'm sorry," when we know that our words have wounded another. I wonder how our world would change. I wonder how people would treat others.

For now, I'll just turn down my hearing aid whenever Florence is around, but I can't help wondering how long it will be until Florence finds herself asking, "What did you say?"

Chapter 29
A PINCH OF LONELINESS

There was another new face today. This time it was not a new cook but a new aide. Elaine's a charming young girl with eyes that sparkle, especially when she talks about her little Tyler, just two years old and already wise enough to challenge Solomon. Elaine dreads the time she must be away from him. She thinks of all the things she is missing and has missed—his first word, his first step, and his first correct attempt at getting the spoon in his mouth. She's a single mom and needs the money to provide food and clothes for Tyler.

Tonight someone else will read Tyler a bedtime story, rock him to sleep and tuck him in. Tonight Elaine walks me to my room and tucks me in instead.

Click! Oh, that sound! I guess that I should feel grateful—I'm in my own room. The click of the lock says I can shut out the world and be in my own secure space surrounded by my family, their smiling faces framed by memories of special occasions in days past. I should feel grateful for my warm, comfortable room, but I feel so alone, so alienated from the world around me.

Loneliness. Didn't someone sing a song once about being lonely in a crowd? I thought that was strange. How could you be lonely surrounded by others? Now I know! I smile. I nod and ask the correct questions about health and weather but I feel so alone. On the days that my batteries die and my hearing aids are not working, I stand like an outsider looking in.

How I long for the friendships of the past when conversations were filled with funny stories about children and interesting information about the neighbors. Friendships that nurtured ideas and dreams on lazy summer days and cozy snowy evenings by the fire.

My friend Alma was always there. If I felt blue, I'd give Alma a call and she could pull back the curtains of my mind and let the sunshine of love flow in. Kay says I'll find new friends here. After all, Alma and most of the others are gone.

"You're doing so well for your age." Do the folks telling me that ever see the loneliness in my eyes? Do they know how much I long for someone to sit and talk with me—really talk without constantly looking at their watch? Do they see the scars on my heart caused by lonely night after lonely night?

Sometimes I envy Ruth. She has just returned from the hospital with a broken arm. Everyone can see the bright pink cast. Everyone takes a minute to ask how she is feeling and to wish her well. The wound on my heart is not visible. Human eyes cannot see the break of my heart nor is there a cast of any color to wrap around it.

Do you know what it feels like to go into a room and sit by yourself while everyone else is talking and laughing? The laughter echoes in your heart like a voice echoing in a tunnel.

I know people don't intentionally mean to ignore you. Often they come into a room and sit in a favorite chair or see someone they know and sit with them. I'm sure that I've done the same thing. It's just different when you're the one experiencing it.

When people pass by you and you're sitting alone, it feels like being the last one picked for the kickball team. I know I shouldn't take it personally and think that something is wrong with me, but just like I did in my teenage years, I head to the bathroom to see if I've sprouted another nose or a third eye.

The image peering back at me assures me that I haven't added any new features to my face, but I do see something else. Just as in those teenage years, I see hollow eyes staring back at me. Eyes filled with loneliness and self-doubt. Each day I wonder, "How can I get through another day?" I might not make it, if it weren't for Ruth...

Chapter 30
LIFE'S DESSERTS

Ruth! What a gift! A few weeks ago, Ruth moved next door bringing with her the sunshine of laughter. I soon learned that she was a creative person who could make masterpieces out of ordinary things. A coffee mug became the base of a beautiful cascading silk flower arrangement. A common white paper plate and some gold ribbon transformed into the best hat of the Hat Day parade. Even creations that would not meet my selective eye were beautiful works of art sprinkled with love. Ruth made her new home and all of us a bit warmer with the glow of her smile.

She also gave me another gift. With Ruth, I could share my family photos and stories without her noticing that I had aged over the years. I could relive special events and happy times. What was most important, I could be myself without having to worry about whether Ruth would accept me or not. I could be me, and Ruth could be Ruth.

I wonder how much of life we spend trying to impress others—trying to be accepted. Often we trade the person we really are for the person we think others want us to be. Perhaps this is a bonus of growing older—learning to accept things and people just as they are.

When Ruth came today, we spent an hour laughing and sharing stories. Stories—the desserts of life. Even when the door closed behind her with that loud click, I noticed that the room seemed brighter and the air usually heavy with loneliness now smelled of seashores and picnics in the woods. Loneliness does not have to be a resident in the home of my heart. Ruth taught me that today. The choice is mine. I can hide from life in the shadows of my room, or share life with those who knock at my door, or who are a call or letter away.

"Grace, it's time for the ladies' tea. Are you coming?"

"Yes, I'll be right there." A cup of tea may be just what I need to help me enjoy life's desserts...

Chapter 31
TWO LUMPS OF MEMORIES

It's called a ladies' tea even though we usually have punch and cookies. Tea is a much better name because tea always makes me think of a warm and comforting beverage. That's what the ladies' tea has become to me—a cup of warmth and comfort from those who gather around the table.

Ginny, the activity director, always has a good topic for us to think about. Usually we talk about families, or childhood memories. Funny school day stories and life's embarrassing moments are always topics sure to brighten our day. I love hearing the stories that the ladies tell. It helps me look behind the smiles or the blank stares of everyday living and see what each is truly feeling.

I certainly looked into hearts today. The topic was how we met our husbands. An interesting topic—but it became much more.

As I looked around the table, I noticed something happen. Eyes suddenly brightened, lips curved into smiles, and years seemed to melt away as our memories carried us back to beautiful times.

Some of the stories were funny: sitting on a swing one day, and running off the next week to become a wife. Some were the "boy next door" stories, or "he was in my class at school," but regardless of the settings, all of the stories had the same ingredients. A magical time when two separate hearts became one. The magic that transformed husbands into heroes who slew the dragons of their days.

Memories. Isn't it strange how memories can both hurt and heal? When Bob first died, memories of him hurt so much. Friends would talk about him, or the kids would remember a special thing that he had said or done, and it would hurt so much that I couldn't even cry. I just wanted to be numb, to not have to feel the pain of the loss. But now years later, gathered with a room filled with other widows, I can tell my story and only feel happiness and gratitude.

Gratitude for a wonderful husband and many years filled with happy days. Gratitude that I have these wonderful memories that become so real now when I talk about them.

Memories that no longer make me numb, but instead bring me new life. Memories that keep Bob alive in my heart, and help me to face each day...

Chapter 32
I LIKE IT

Today I was really bored. How do you know? I went to the daily Bingo game! Bingo is my least favorite activity. In fact it ranks right up there with a trip to the dentist and a case of the flu. But today I just couldn't find anything to do. Turning to CNN and watching the daily news depressed me. Trying to write to my cousin frustrated me as my eyes refused to focus on the paper. Even my hearing was distorting the music on my tape player, so in desperation, I opened my door and headed to the daily treasure hunt of letters and numbers.

Arriving at the activity room I found a chair in the corner nearest the doorway. My game plan was to escape when I could no longer stand the torture. I dutifully took a card and the red plastic markers handed to me and waited to be miserable.

The activity director's voice boomed out the letter and number. Her voice sounded harsh since she had to scream out the letters and numbers to be heard. Even then, she had to repeat for those dear souls who thought there was going to be a B70! Pathetic you may say from the sidelines, but let me tell you what I saw happen right before my eyes.

I saw Jane win the game with her eyes closed! Pretty amazing, right. It would be if somehow Jane had sensed the right letter and number without even looking, but that is not what happened. You see, Jane was asleep!

She won because Sophie sat next to her and gently placed the marker on the right spot as it was called. I thought that was kind, and then I stopped to really look and listen.

"You have it, John."
"Here's B12, Ed. Let me cover it for you."
"Look, she has Bingo. Call it out, Myrtle."

No one seemed to be interested in his or her own card. Instead they were more interested in the letters and numbers of the person sitting beside them or across from them. Winning was not the name of the game. Helping was.

It didn't matter that eyes closed and markers fell lazily out of one's hand. There was always a helping hand ready to take over—to be the eyes and hands of another.

When someone thought that 70 could be in the B column, no one ridiculed. Instead they just reminded that the number was B12.

B12. I always thought of that as a vitamin my body needed, but today I found that B12 was a vitamin my soul needed. A reminder that in this game of life, winning is not as important as helping the players.

You know maybe there is more to this game then I thought. Maybe I should make it part of my daily routine like my prune juice cocktail...

Chapter 33
THE PRUNE JUICE COCKTAIL

My morning routine now includes a prune juice cocktail. I drink it not because I enjoy it, but because it helps things move more smoothly.

Today when Betty served it to me, I realized that she needed life to move more smoothly for her too.

Dragging herself into work after a sleepless night, Betty told me about the phone call. The phone call everyone dreads—the one from the police. There had been an accident. Betty's heart skipped a beat as she learned that her elderly father had been in an automobile accident. She had rushed to the hospital, relieved to find her father alive, but worried that the cuts and bruises were hiding more serious injuries. Now he was in the hospital and Betty had a list of phone calls that had to be made. But instead of calling, she was serving prune juice cocktails. Despite her worries, Betty needed this job to meet her family's needs.

Her questions of, "Why me?" and, "How much more can I take?" gave voice to the burdens weighing down upon her shoulders.

It would be easy for me to say to Betty, "Things could be worse." I could point out that her father could have been killed. I could have reminded her of others consuming bitter dishes of life—victims of disease or natural disasters or terrorists. But for Betty those things would still not seem as bad as what she is facing now. When our plate is filled with personal difficulties, we can only feel the stabbing pain of those hurts.

Strange isn't it? I'm the one residing in a facility that is supposed to assist me with living, but this morning the one who comes to help me needs the help. Then again maybe it's not so strange. Isn't that what life is all about? Helping each other.

So as my hand reaches out for the prune juice, I'll let it linger a little longer on Betty's. I'll listen without offering advice. I'll just listen, so Betty's cares and worries can escape her heart and flit through the sunlight in my room. I'll tell her that I'm sorry for all she is facing, and tell her that I'll pray for her to have the strength to get through this day and face another.

But perhaps I too should ask God the same question. "Why me?" Why did you choose me, God, to be here when Betty needed someone to share her burden? Could my answer be found in reheating the main course of life?

Chapter 34
REHEATING THE MAIN COURSE

This morning I was sure that my brain had been fried over night. I arrived at breakfast ready to greet my bowl of oatmeal and the new day. Instead I was greeted with, "Grace, you are wearing one black and one blue shoe."

There was a day not long ago when those words would have sent me scurrying back to the safety of my room. Slamming the door behind me, I would have stirred up a new batch of fritters to remind me that my mental abilities were failing, and that soon I would be helpless, unaware of what I was doing, and a worry to my family.

Today, however, I greeted the words with a chuckle, and soon everyone was laughing as I added, "I like a little color in my life." (Of course this wouldn't have happened if I had worn my red shoes to breakfast!) Everyone started the day with a smile, but I started mine with much more—the knowledge that I'm able to reheat the main course of life.

At last I am losing some of my fears and self-consciousness about growing older. I say "some," because there are still days that I can't face reality—days that my self-confidence stays in bed and refuses to get dressed. But those days are fewer as I've learned to accept myself at this stage in life.

Ah, the stages of life. Growing up is never easy. Children want to cling to those days of carefree play instead of beginning the rigors of a school routine. Adolescents struggle to find their independence in the midst of dependency. Adults too must grow up to the reality that once again, if we live long enough, we will depend on others for help with basic needs.

There seems to be a revolving door on the kitchen of life taking us back to where we first began to cook the broth of life. Yet, there's a unique beauty in reheating this main course and in tasting anew the love of caring and receiving.

In my ninety years, I've added many spoonfuls of losses to my broth. Pictures remind me of the loss of loved ones; the mirror, of the loss of youth; my walker, of the loss of independence. But now those losses are softened with the awareness that I have also lost the things that for years have robbed me of my appetite for a richer life. I now realize that each day is indeed a gift that needs to be opened with care and genuine anticipation of something wonderful.

I have lost the desire to look in the mirror and wish someone else were looking back at me. Instead of looking for flaws and tiny imperfections, I accept the face that is mine. I'm even beginning to see the beauty of the face framed with the wrinkles of a life well lived.

Today the activity director wanted to take my picture for the hall bulletin board. My hair looked like it had been in a tropical storm. In my younger days, I would have refused to let my picture be taken, but today I smiled broadly. For you see, I'm now old enough not to care about what I look like as long as I'm not in a casket. In my own eyes, I've finally grown old enough to be beautiful.

"You look good for your age" is a statement I hear a lot. Wonder what that means? How is a ninety-year-old woman supposed to look? Is there a Dr. Spock for the elderly that tells how one should look and act at ninety? What do they see when they say I look "good for my age?"

Well, lately I have come to realize that I do look good for my age. I look like a warrior who has fought the battles of life and lived to tell about it. The battle scars of wrinkles and white hair may make you think that the fight was fierce, and at times it was. But what you can't see is the reason for the sparkle in my eyes and the grin on my face.

I have lost the desire to be always perfect in the eyes of everyone. Admitting mistakes has even opened the door to conversations as others share similar experiences. I realize that I can be the person I really am instead of the person I think people would like me to be.

Worrying over my loss of remembering clouds my vision for seeing the new opportunities that today brings. I have accepted the fact that it's OK not to remember every detail of my last ninety years. My friends don't remember them either.

Most of all I have learned to accept myself and to laugh away the little things that in my earlier days would have tied me in a knot of inferiority. I've learned to face my losses and look for a blessing in each of them. That's not always easy. Some days, I feel like I'm on a roller coaster—climbing the hills of acceptance one moment and plunging into the depths of doubt in the next. Strangely, when the ride is over, I'm still able to stand tall and know that each day needs to be lived to its fullest without looking back or ahead.

I've learned that life is a journey, a beautiful journey if we choose to take the time to help another along the way. For in helping another we again are reminded of the many blessings we have been given.

Yes, I've tasted many dishes of living in my ninety years. Accepting myself has been one that I've had to acquire a taste for, and yet perhaps that dish holds the answer to how one ages gracefully and how one gracefully treats the aged.

Perhaps in my test kitchen of life, I really have been following a recipe for living and aging...

Chapter 35
THE RECIPE

All my life I've followed the recipes of others to create thousands of dishes for family and friends. Now in the waning years of my life, I realize that the best recipe I own is not one from the family treasure house. It's not from the countless recipes that I collected in books, cut from papers and glossy magazine pages or scribbled on the back of a scrap of whatever material happened to be close at hand. My best recipe is one that I have written myself with the blood, sweat and tears of living. It goes like this:

RECIPE FOR AGING

Into the pot of life carefully measure heaping cups of love.

Remove any irritating traits that may come packaged with your family and friends, and carefully blend in patience and encouragement.

Add an appreciation of the beauty found in the world around you. Take time to notice feathery clouds and crimson sunsets. Listen to the anthems of birds and the symphony of crickets.

Mix heaping measures of joy to everyday chores and cherish the memories of a job well done.

When doubts, fears and anger spill into life's broth, quickly strain them out and add large amounts of faith, courage and forgiveness.

If the broth becomes thin or bitter whip in courage and acceptance.

Use this broth of life as the main ingredient for a variety of dishes to be shared in the banquet hall of life.

Savor to the very last drop.

"Grace, it's time for dinner. We're trying a new recipe tonight."

"Oh, really? Well, I have a recipe that you might like to try..."

REFLECTION QUESTIONS

Chapter 1

In today's culture that puts so much emphasis on looking young, how do you feel about your wrinkles?

What things about your life are told by your wrinkles?

What's a favorite recipe or dish of your childhood? Who was the person that made it? Was it made at a certain time or for a certain occasion?

What's your comfort food?

Do you have any "recipe friends?" Why have they become special to you?

Do your "recipe friends" tell you anything about yourself?

Chapter 2

Grace talks about the magic in her stages of life. Think about your childhood, teenage years, and adulthood. What magic was in those years for you?

What are some of the daily routines that bring your contentment or brought your contentment in the past?

How do you feel when a friend gets sick or dies?

Think about a time when you made a difficult move in your life.

Chapter 3

Describe a "moving day stew" that you remember tasting in your life.

What do you consider the hardest part of moving?

What things do you think are the hardest to give up in downsizing?

Can you name something in your life that you wish you had kept? Why is that object now important to you?

Think of an object that you would keep in your family.

Describe a house in your life that was like a special friend.

What was a move that turned out to be a good move for you?

What is the hardest loss that you have had to deal with?

Think of some things that were helpful to you when you have experienced grief that might help another?

Can you name something good that has come out of a loss?

Chapter 4

Reflect on a time when you felt like you were living in a "pressure cooker."

How do you think making a move to an assisted living facility can be made more comfortable?

Chapter 5

Do you think it's a good idea to move closer to family even if the move means leaving your community and friends?

What are some suggestions for making friends when you have moved to a new home?

Chapter 6

What are good things to talk about when meeting strangers?

What can you do when a situation seems frightening?

Chapter 7

1. Have you ever felt like you were "drowning in the fog of medication?"

What can be done to prevent becoming over medicated?

What does "quality of life" mean to you?

Chapter 8

What are some things that you enjoy doing?

What are some things that do not bring you enjoyment?

Do you have a comfort zone? Does it limit you from trying new things?

Chapter 9

How would you answer Grace's questions of "How would you fill your days if your world suddenly shrank to one room? How would you fill the minutes in the hours, and the hours in the day?"

If your life was in a locked box, what would be in the box?

Chapter 10

What do you think is scary about making new friends?

What does Grace really mean when she says she is often not strong enough to get to the other side of the door?

Chapter 11

What does Grace mean when she says," Looking through photo albums is like attending a banquet of life?"

If all your photos were lost, what would you miss most?

Chapter 12

How do you feel when you look in the mirror?

What about growing older bothers you?

What makes you laugh?

Chapter 13

What are some ways that you can encourage others?

Did you meet anyone today who needs to be encouraged?

Think of someone who does a job that usually does not get appreciated. How could you show that person that you appreciate what he or she does?

What does Grace mean when she says, "Wrinkles are reminders that we are aging from within with a beauty that allows us the time and patience to offer love to others?"

Chapter 14

What are your favorite daydreams?

Do you think it is painful to dream of the past?

Grace describes dreams as " visitors arriving with the invitation to return to the special places and people that flavored days with contentment and joy." How would you describe dreams?

Chapter 15

Why do you think it is hard to forgive someone who has hurt you?

How does one take the first step in mending a broken relationship?

Do you think Jean's death was a tragedy?

Chapter 16

When you read about Dan, did you feel sorry for him, or wish you were more like him?

How does one "look at people through the eyes of the heart?"

Chapter 17

Do you have anything that reminds you of another time in your life?

Did you ever buy something impractical? How did it make you feel?

How has your world changed?

Grace wants others to know "my spirit is still sturdy even if the container in which it is housed needs some repairs." How does one help others to understand that?

Do you have "red shoes" in your life that stand for your independence?

Chapter 18

Have you ever had an experience like Grace where something that should have brought you contentment didn't?

Think of a time when "contentment was sloshing in front of your eyes and you were blinded to its image."

Chapter 19

What was dinnertime like at your house when you were growing up?

If you had a magic salt shaker what would it produce?

What is the worst meal that you remember?

Chapter 20

What do the words "right away" mean to you? Can you think of a time when they meant something else to another person with whom you were dealing?

What does Grace mean when she says, " time is not always measured by
the seconds and minutes and hours of the clock?"

3. Name some ways that you have grown more patient with age.

Chapter 21

Think of a time when you were hesitant about complaining because you felt someone might become angry.

How does one correct a situation without causing bad feelings?

What is the difference between complaining and correcting a situation?

Chapter 22

Do you agree with Grace that if we live long enough, we come "full circle?"

What do "older kids" need?

Chapter 23

Describe how you feel about pain?

How do you feel about the aging of your body?

What do you think Grace means when she says, "At times it seems like my pain is not about what I eat, but what eats me."

Do you think pain is ever related to fear?

Chapter 24

How would you answer Grace's question, "Do you make fritters too?"

What are the fears that we have at different stages of our lives?

What are some of the "little things" in life that are important to people?

What little things can you do to brighten someone's day?

Chapter 25

What are your cravings?

Can you think of a time when you felt invisible?

If you had been Grace at the doctor's office would you have remained invisible?

How can we show more respect to the elderly?

Chapter 26

Give some examples of ways that we all want to be noticed.

What is hard to accept about yourself?

What is the hardest thing that you have noticed about growing older?

What are some new things that you have learned as you age?

Chapter 27

For parents and grandparents:

How are your experiences of being a parent and grandparent similar or different from Grace's experiences?

For everyone:

Think of a special child that you know. What has that child helped you to see that you had not seen before?

Chapter 28

What are some problems you have had with not hearing well?

Think of something that you heard that you wished you had not heard.

Give an example of words that encourage.

Give an example of words that discourage.

Chapter 29

Describe a time when you felt lonely in a crowd.

How does it feel to be ignored?

Can you think of a way to be more aware of the wounds on another's heart?

Chapter 30

Describe a special friend of yours.

Do you agree with Grace that we spend a lot of our lives trying to impress others?

Explain what Grace means when she says, "Loneliness does not have to be a resident in the home of my heart."

Give an example of "hiding from life."

Chapter 31

Tell how you met your mate or a special person in your life.

How do memories both hurt or heal?

Share a special memory of your mate or another special person in your life.

Chapter 32

What did Grace learn from the Bingo game?

How important do you think winning is in the game of life?

Can you think of a time when helping another was more important than winning?

Chapter 33

Think of a time when you asked the question, "Why me?"

How do you feel about Grace's statement that life is about helping others?

What did Grace really do for Betty?

Chapter 34

Can you think of something that bothered you when you were young that does not bother you now?

What stage of life do you think is most difficult? Why?

What does Grace mean when she says that she has "grown old enough to be beautiful?"

What does "looking good for your age" mean to you?

Can you think of any ways that you are "reheating the main course of your life?"

Chapter 35

What does Grace's recipe show that she has learned about life?

If you wrote a recipe for aging, what would it include?

Printed in the United States
83728LV00007B/13-30/A

9 781424 177370